I0436212

What Shoes Are You Wearing Today?
A *Man's* Walk with Lupus

A Memoir

ALLEN MENDRIN

Life isn't about waiting for the storm to pass; it's about learning to dance in the rain

- Author Unknown

What Shoes Are You Wearing Today?
A *Man's* Walk with Lupus

CONTENTS

CHAPTER 12

FUTURE OUTLOOK FOR LUPUS PATIENTS

ACKNOWLEDGEMENTS

PROLOGUE

Have you ever had to prepare for an interview? If you have, you may have practiced responding to questions in the mirror, had a friend pose possible interview questions or had them critique your responses to questions. You may be the type of person who needs to write out what you might possibly say if asked a possible interview question. I happen to be all the above!

My interview was scheduled for Monday, but for some reason it was cancelled and the interviewer asked if I was up for an over the phone interview. I agreed and the appointment was set for later on that week.

By Tuesday I was back in the hospital. I was accustom to the emergency room procedure, I knew what floor I was going to be on and I, unfortunately, was familiar with the doctors and nurses. This Lupus disease was affecting me in a way I could not yet control. It was playing me like a puppet on a string. It had me in its vise grip and had no intentions of easing up. All I was able to do was take my medications, look out my window at the blue skies, check out the surfers with my binoculars and hope my body recovered enough so I could put on my hospital shoes and make an exit.

After a couple of days of the resting, waiting, watching, praying and anything else I could possible do to pass the time; it was time for my interview. How could I possibly have this interview over the phone with all the screams of beeping coming from my heart monitor, blood pressure, and oxygen monitors? Not to mention, the doctors, nurses, nursing assistants, phlebotomists, respiratory therapists, lunch personnel, and many others who at anytime could walk into my hospital room and cause for me to vindicate myself to the interviewer.

My time management was critical. I had to plan my treatments around my interview time. I had to literarily make sure I could breathe long enough to make it through my interview. I had to make sure all the sounds of the machines were on silent, oh yeah and make sure I remembered all my preparation questions and answers. This was going to be more difficult than I thought.

The phone rings. I recognize my possible future employer's phone number. My hospital room (which I converted into my personal office with papers spread all around me as I laid in the gurney) is absent of beeping and caring personnel. The interview starts. As I conquer the questions asked, I can't help but think of how this might be the first hospital/gurney phone interview ever. (Although a hospital gurney is a rare place for an interview, there is probably someone out there who has experienced what I had experienced.) If the ones asking the questions only knew where I was, what I have gone through to prepare for their phone call and what I had to do to prepare myself. I have gone through so much just to prepare the environment. I was meticulous in covering "everything under the sun" as best as possible to make where I am unnoticeable. To think of how one typically would prepare for an interview and compare it to how I had to prepare for this interview was fascinating to me.

Just as I had to prepare for this interview, I needed to prepare my life for this new disease. I had to strategically plan when I was going to take my medications, how I was going to get from point A to point B, and sometimes how I was going to get out of bed! This disease wasn't going to allow for me to take my everyday walks of life for granted. I was going to have a plan of action from here on out. Lupus is my new employer, I work for Lupus. Will I ever be my own boss? Will I ever make my own schedule? Will Lupus ever let me have the control I once took for granted?

INTRODUCTION

A MAN WITH LUPUS

Lupus, me! I was 28 years old, fit before my diagnosis and never in the world would I expect to have something I couldn't get rid of. I had things to do, I was an educator in need of doing my job and I didn't want to be confined to the hospital. The diagnosis came as a shock to me. I didn't expect this in my life! I didn't imagine Lupus affecting and attacking my vital organs either. (*I'll explain these symptoms later.*) The shoes of choice were now chosen for me. The shoes on the front cover of this book are known as my "hospital shoes." My shoes and I kept good company over the next month.

I am, and will forevermore be, from this point on, a *MAN* battling *Systemic Lupus Erythematosus, (*SLE.) Specifically, Lupus is attacking my joints, my kidneys (Diffuse Proliferative Lupus Nephritis, Class IV,) and my lungs (Acute Alveolar Hemorrhaging.) There are an estimated (2 to 2.5 million people in the US who are affected with Lupus. (LupusFoundation.org) One out of about every 10 are males and I happen to be one of them.

I was diagnosed in January 2009 and have since been on a mission to find as much information about this autoimmune disease as possible. To say the least, it has been difficult to find research and information pertaining to men and the current conditions I now embrace. I wanted to write this book to help individuals who are experiencing the same conditions, emotions, attitudes, beliefs, struggles, and successes I am going through. To my Lupus friends, fathers, mothers, sisters, uncles, aunts, grandmas and grandpas with lupus or know of someone who has lupus….. This is for you!

CHAPTER 1

THE SHOES YOU WEAR

The shoes a person puts on everyday can reveal a lot about what he or she does or is about to do throughout the events of their upcoming day. Some might put on dress shoes, maybe because they are going into the office or business workforce. Others may put on athletic shoes because they are on their way to the gym or its "Casual Friday." Some may put on flip flops to go to the beach or the lake to relax. Whatever the occasion, the shoes you put on can say a lot about the events that might unfold throughout your day.

What about people who don't put on shoes in the morning? These people might be staying home for the day, they might not have somewhere to go so there is no need for shoes, or they may have other plans to do before they put their shoes on. My story involves my shoe acquaintance of slippers! Slippers! Yes, I have a particular pair of slippers I have come to endear. They have inspired me because they are sometimes the shoes I need to wear to get me to where I need to go and back.

My "hospital slippers" as I call them, are only worn to and from the hospital. They stay outside my door if I am not in the hospital and if they are absent from their stationed position it's because I am in the hospital. I would prefer to always have them just outside my house door, but sometimes the fortunes in one's life are not choices they would choose. I've contemplated throwing my hospital slippers away, but every time I go in-and-out of my door, they remind me of the events I have been through in my life and they give me encouragement of what I have accomplished! I am glad to have my slippers and fortunate not to have thrown them away!

The picture on the front cover shows my hospital slippers. They were given to me as a gift by my sister Susan in December 2008, just as I was starting to feel my first symptoms of joint pain. My hospital slippers are warm and comforting and hold much sentimental value because they were used to walk some very hard and difficult steps.

CHAPTER 2

WHO AM I?

My name is Allen. I am 28 years old. I am a MALE living, breathing, walking, running, and battling Lupus. I grew up in Fresno, California. I have 3 siblings; Stephanie, Susan, and Michael. I have an awesome mother Carolyn, who is a major rock and foundation in my life. I grew up on the farm where we raised sheep, cows, pigeons, and ducks, grew vegetables, and swung from ropes onto bails of broken hay like wild Indians. Looking back, I remember always being dirty and muddy because of the snakes, lizards, bees, and leprechaun hunts I would adventure on as a kid growing up on the farm.

My college years were spent at California State University, Fresno (CSUF) where I majored in Science. I also participated on the track team where I threw the javelin and high jumped. I had ambitions of becoming a dentist, but I had always loved to work with kids and taught at Sunday school throughout my college years. One day a friend encouraged me to get into substitute teaching and took the necessary steps to do so. It was my first day of subbing (Kindergarten) where I kept feeling the thoughts and emotions of the clear direction of becoming an educator. I continued my education at CSUF, where I earned a Bachelor of Science in Biology and minored in Philosophy. I also obtained my teaching credential. My first teaching position was kindergarten, oh what patients that taught me!

In 2005, I married my very own angel, Nicole and she truly is my better half. We have been married for four years now and currently have no kids, but I was lucky enough to adopt her little dog, Lola. (She is a feisty, but a very loveable Chihuahua!)

My religious perspective is that I love the Lord and put Him first in all areas of my life. I often pray and ask Him to keep my heart, ears, and eyes open through this battling process so that I understand what He is trying to teach me.

Nicole and I relocated to Southern California in the summer of 2005. We relocated to the beach because I liked the sand and she loved the water so we compromised and ended up at a wonderful beach called Sunset Beach. I currently teach middle school Science and have recently earned my administrative credential and my wife is working through the nursing program. My life is good, except when I when I have to put on the shoes I didn't think I would ever have to wear!

CHAPTER 3

LUPUS, WHAT'S LUPUS?

Lupus is an *Autoimmune Disease*, which turns the bodies' normal immune system against itself, at times. There is no cure for Lupus. Doctors and researchers don't know why people get Lupus. It is called Lupus because some forms of Lupus affect the skin in an appearance which looks like individuals were bitten or scratched by wolves. Thus, Lupus in Latin means "wolf." (http://www.sjlupus.org/info.html) There are an estimated 16,000 new cases of Lupus diagnosed each year and the particular age range at diagnosis is between 18 and 55 years of age. Women are ten to fifteen times more likely to get Lupus than men. Kids can also get Lupus for unknown reasons. There is research which concludes family members can have five to twelve percent chance of acquiring Lupus. Newborns, of mothers with lupus, can have up 5% chance of developing Lupus. (http://www.lupus.org) Individuals, *like me*, can acquire Lupus without having any other relative or family member indicating signs or having any other *Autoimmune Diseases* like Lupus!

Lupus has three different forms: d*rug-induced lupus, Discoid Lupus, and Systemic Lupus Erythematosus.*

1. *Drug-induced Lupus* is caused by specific ingested chemicals, such as medications.

2. Lupus only of the skin is called *Discoid Lupus*. This form of Lupus is sometimes traceable by altering patches of skin color which may be red, dry, flakey, or scaly.

3. *Systemic Lupus Erythematosus* (SLE) is a disease that can involve and affect every organ in the body. *Systemic* means "general." (This is the type of Lupus I have.)

As stated previously, there is no underlining reason of why individuals get Lupus. There is also no cure for Lupus. There are some possible suggestions of what may trigger Lupus to take action in individuals; these suggestions include: certain genes are "triggered" to become activated in one's body (although it is not considered a genetic disease), the sun and defective suppressor cells (which help the body regulate, check and prevent the body's immune system from overreacting.)

The signs and symptoms can be different patient to patient. In other words, no two cases are alike. Some of these symptoms are more frequent or sudden than others and some come and go as they please. The signs and symptoms may be similar in males and females. People with Lupus may have the following symptoms:

- Fatigue
- Fever
- Weight loss or gain
- Joint pain, stiffness and swelling
- Butterfly-shaped rash (malar rash) on the face that covers the cheeks and bridge of the nose
- Skin lesions that appear or worsen with sun exposure
- Mouth sores
- Hair loss (alopecia)
- Fingers and toes that turn white or blue when exposed to cold or during stressful periods (Reynaud's phenomenon)
- Shortness of breath
- Chest pain
- Dry eyes
- Easy bruising

- Anxiety
- Depression
- Memory loss

(http://www.mayoclinic.com)

CHAPTER 4

MY DIAGNOSIS

So I have Lupus! It is affecting my joints (to the point of me having to use crutches at times,) my Kidneys (Diffuse Proliferative Lupus Nephritis, Class IV) and my lungs (Alveolar Hemorrhaging.) Talk about scary! One day I'm dunking a basketball and the next I can hardly walk or breath. I was a division 1 track athlete in college and running and physical fitness has always been a top priority and not being able to do what I once was able to do, is scary.

I started noticing joint pain in December of 2008. My wife and I went home for Christmas to visit our family and enjoy the holidays with our friends. One morning a friend invited me to play basketball at a local fitness club. It sounded fun, so I agreed and went to the gym to play a little early morning basketball. Throughout the first game I remember having difficulty breathing and both my feet hurt badly. I had to sit out the next game to rest my feet, catch my breath and take my shoes off. I resumed playing after resting a game and went home.

Playing basketball, running about three miles per week, surfing, working out, biking and playing softball were all common activities I partook in throughout, what was for me at the time, a normal week. So, I didn't think anything of it other than maybe I was getting a little ill or I didn't warm-up enough. Speaking of getting sick, I (for as long as I can remember) typically got sick once a year. I mean sick like both of my ends having serious action! This would typically last 2-3 days and because of the yearly routine for many years of my life, I would not worry about getting sick from that point on for about another year. Other than that, a sniffle here and there would periodically come about, but never anything major.

It's so interesting for me to recall all this information as clearly as I do. As I spent time in the hospital, as you will read, I kept a journal, wrote down thoughts, prayers, and time frames. I just wanted to do my best so in the case any of you having these symptoms, you can get treatment as soon as possible and have a good indication of what to expect, if you know of a person going through the battles I have gone through.

That night, around Christmas, I was sitting in my mom's rocking chair. By the way, I love to rock, I feel so at ease rocking, it comforts me, relaxes me, soothes me and probably makes me look foolish every time I enter a room with a rocking chair and dash straight for it. I have always rocked and will always rock. I am rocking right now as I type these words. Okay let's put it this way, if I couldn't be in a rocking chair for a long period of time I would go insane. If you want to seriously mess with me, take away my rocking chair!

Anyway, back to that night of visiting my mom sitting in the rocking chair. I noticed my body was feeling uncomfortable. I had slight pain basically from head to toe. It was in my: ankles, back, elbows, wrists, fingers, neck, and mostly knees. I didn't think anything of it because earlier in the day, after basketball, I painted my mother's bathroom and one could expect to be sore after a vigorous activity of that sort. I took some Tylenol and went to bed. The next morning I had very little pain, still assuming it was from my painting exhibition, I went on enjoying friends and family for the next couple of days and my wife and I went home.

Over the next couple of weeks I noticed my body to be "more than normal" fatigued or sluggish to say the least and that my joints were achy. I am a teacher and at this point in time I would: go home and have to take a nap, get up and have enough energy to make it to dinner. I thought to myself that this feeling was "interesting." I decided to stopped running, working out and all other activities for a week so that my exhausted body could rest.

I decided to make a doctor's appointment and scheduled a general physical. My last physical was August 28th 2008 where my blood work was assessed and all areas of my health and blood work were in excellent condition. I was fine during the doctor's visit in August. On January 13th 2009 I scheduled another physical with my primary doctor to conduct a check-up and discuss why I was feeling fatigued and why my joints were slightly hurting. He scheduled blood work to be drawn and a urine sample. The results came back abnormal!

My primary doctor sent me to a Rheumatologist. He said some of my blood work came back "out of range" and he knew of a good doctor to discuss the results with me. To be honest with you, I didn't even know who or what a Rheumatologist was, but boy did I find out! My Rheumatologist scheduled me for a procedure called a 24-hour urine collection. Apparently, according to my latest urine analysis, the protein in my urine came back high and this test would further help determine what specific range my excreting protein was in. Just as this may be new to you or a loved one, this was all new to me. When I asked about what I was going to be doing for the 24-hour urine collection, she explained "I just needed to collect my urine for a period of 24-hours." I figured that was the task because of the name of the procedure, but I was more so wondering along the lines of how I was going to do this at school and pondering that the task wasn't going to be that easy.

I went down to the lab, which was in the same office building as the doctor, to get my 24-hour urine container. It was brown, plastic and reminded me of a football. I listened to the instructions and went on my way. Yep, my container and I were going to be side-by-side and hand-in-hand for the next day. The next day just happened to be a Thursday and I teach at the middle school level!

The next day I was not allowed to use the toilet if I had to pee. I had to relieve myself in a cup and pour it into the football (24-hour urine container). The 24-hour urine container holds up to 2 liters. After my first deposit, I was thinking, I should have gotten two of them! I started at 7am. This was fine because I was at home. I needed a way to conceal my "football" from the students and the staff. To make matters even more challenging, the container had to be kept in the refrigerator the entire 24-hours. I decided to take the container, tie it up in two plastic bags and conceal it in my gym bag. Needless to say, after a day of going to the refrigerator, untying my "football", peeing in a cup, transferring my urine and people asking me what was in the bag for lunch; I made it through the day. The most exciting part of the experience was the appreciation of just simply being able to use the toilet to pee without the hassle of collecting it. Just that experience alone puts a different perspective on people and their limitations. This experience allowed me to appreciate my capabilities even more.

My next visit was to the Rheumatologist. I remember sitting in the Rheumatologists office on the patient's gurney, you know the one that is covered in a thin paper which either tears or makes a thunderous crunching sound every time you move, looking at my wife waiting impatiently for the doctor to enter the room. Finally, when the Rheumatologist arrived, she went over the blood work results. The doctor stated that because of the different areas of my blood work being out of range, the fatigue, the high protein and blood amounts in the 24-hour urine and because of the joint pain; she suspected I had Lupus. As my wife and I sat there tearing up, the doctor explained to us what Lupus was, what parts of the body it affects, how to treat it and how to cope with it.

I have always been an optimistic person and will always be and after hearing what the doctor had to say, I immediately asked the question of "Am I going to die?" The doctor looked shocked I would ask such a direct question and stated that *some* people live with Lupus for a long time and have full life expectancies. I posed the question as a joke to break the ice in the intense room, but to be honest I was encouraged with her answer because I knew that I was that *someone.*

I remember thinking, after we left the doctor's office, that I was 28 years old, fit before this and never in the world would I expect to have a disease I couldn't get rid of. I had things to do in my life! I remember thinking that I was a husband, I was a teacher, and I didn't want to have Lupus.

I was now faced with a new challenge in my life. I didn't know it at the time, but this challenge in my life developed for a reason and different perspectives, hopes and dreams were developed because of this occurrence. The shoes I have been wearing for the last 28 years of my life were in the midst of changing.

Joint pain was present for me, but the Lupus was also affecting my kidneys. This was determined from my 24-hour urine analysis. Days following the Rheumatologists visit, I went to the kidney doctor and we set-up an appointment to have a kidney biopsy. This type of biopsy consist of the doctor applying local anesthesia on my lower back, sticking a long needle into where one of my kidneys was located, (when Systematic Lupus is occurring it effects both organs, not just one, according to my doctors and it didn't matter which kidney was biopsied on,) and extracting kidney samples. The biopsy was scheduled and we were waiting for the appointment, but we never made it to that day because I was admitted to the hospital days before the appointment and stayed there days after.

CHAPTER 5
THE HOSPITAL VISITS

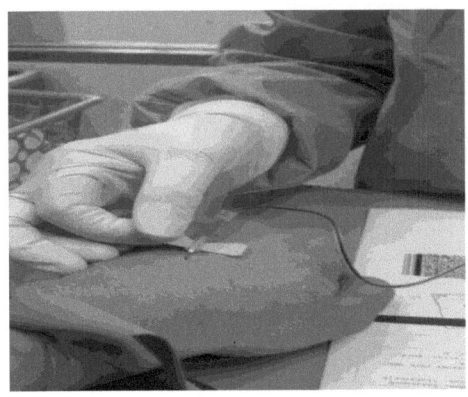

My First Hospital Stay

Hospitals are a great place to work, but never a fun place to stay especially if you don't want to be there. Yes, the food was good (choice cut steaks and mashed potatoes) and the assistance was nice, but it's very difficult to actually rest in the hospital.

For the past week I was running a high fever of 102 degrees and having night chills. Throughout that week I called the doctor's office and she told me to take Tylenol. That wasn't helping with the fever. The fever would come and go. I called the doctor's office once more and asked if the severe chills were a dilemma to be concerned with and the doctor stated "It's was due to the Lupus and if the fever went up to 104 degrees it would call for medical attention." There have been many times the doctors explain why situations were happening to me with the answer of, *"It's caused by the Lupus or the Lupus is in direct relationship to why you feel this way."*

This is frustrating sometimes because there is still so much not known about Lupus, but research is progressing and the more people share their stories and make connections, the better understood it will become.

The doctor told me to have some blood work done and I headed into the office. During my blood work visit, I literally ran into my doctor in the elevator. She asked me to go to her office where she checked me out. After examining me she advised me to check myself into the hospital because of my continuous chills and high fever of 102 degrees.

I called my wife, told her the news and not to worry and drove myself to the emergency room. As I waited, which felt like days, (actually hours) I finally got admitted into my patient room for the first time. I was impressed with the room because it had a great view of the ocean. (Hoag Hospital is an exceptional hospital that is known for their superb patient care and excellent views of the Pacific Ocean.)

Once admitted, the doctors started me on the first round of high dose Prednisone (100 mg). It is given intravenously and is used to suppress the immune system, which was causing my Lupus to flare up, which was causing my high fever and causing my severe chills. The Prednisone, which I will discuss in more detail about and its side effects later, was the first of three treatments.

FLARE UP

This is a great time to talk about what flare ups are. With Lupus, symptoms can be quite vast. Some people have just the joint pain, some have skin problems and others (like me) have internal organ problems with joint pain. My first "flare up" consisted of severe joint pain (knees mostly) and my kidneys became inflamed. This inflammation of my kidneys caused large amount of protein and blood to be excreted into the urine. Many people are different in how they respond to their personal flare ups and these situations are often the worst times for Lupus patients. There are many opinions out there on why individuals flare up, but there are no known certainties. From the research I gathered, flare ups seem to vary individual to individual.

The doctors suggested since I was in the hospital I should have my kidney biopsy. I thought it was a good idea too. The biopsy was more intriguing of a procedure then hurtful. The biopsy allowed doctors to classify the kidneys based on a I, II, III, IV, or V classification scale with class I being the least severe or mildest and class V being the most severe. The classification level would allow the doctors to properly treat the kidneys and Lupus. I was told the results would take weeks to get and the doctor would call me when the results were ready.

Along with the prednisone, kidney biopsy, and other medications pumped into my body, I also had a chest x-ray (to check for Pneumonia, which came back negative) and CT scan of my chest cavity. The CT scan showed that my spleen was enlarged and that, of course, was *"from the Lupus."*

As I finished up my second day in the hospital and gathered my belongings, I was administered my second round of prednisone and was cleared for discharge. I left my truck at the hospital and my wife and I agreed to pick it up in the morning because the Prednisone had the tendency to have side effects, which fogs my mind heavily. My side effects from prednisone also include: dizziness and extreme agitation. So, driving at this point was out of the question. Thank goodness my loving wife was by-my-side and drove me home. At home, I was ordered to take 60 mg of Prednisone and I would be on it for the next 2.5 months.

A quick story about how Prednisone effects my mind is that on one night, at dinner, I was feeling "not so calm", to say the least! My wife made us dinner which consisted of chicken, vegetables, and mashed potatoes. I made my plate and decided the mashed potatoes needed gravy. I haven't had gravy with mash potatoes, at my house, in over 3 years! Why I wanted gravy, I didn't know why, I just wanted them! My food got cold, because I decided I wanted and needed to find it in the pantry and heat it up. I then layered the thick gravy over the cold potatoes. As I was walking to the table I noticed that I hadn't put salt onto the newly dressed potatoes. With me being very frustrated and agitated (at no one in particular) I took the salt and threw it across the room. What was I thinking? How childish was I acting? Its gravy! Really, salt put me over the edge? Actually, it did! My wife and I look back on that day and laugh because that wasn't a normal reaction for me and we know it was without doubt caused by the side effects of the Prednisone. Later, I split open my big toe, blood everywhere, retrieving the salt shaker I tossed. It found it's was under a heavy cedar chest which I pulled out to viciously and caught my big toe. I guess that will teach me to throw the salt around!

After the salt throwing night, I had to go back to the outpatient center for my last IV treatment of Prednisone. The treatment facility, again, had to poke me to start an IV. This time the IV couldn't be started because my blood vessels couldn't be found. They tried four different times! The nurses said my IV wouldn't start do to the previous steroid treatments, apparently it effects ones veins by constricting them. The nurses brought in their secret weapon, an IV specialist! On one shot, *ha that's funny*; she was able to start the IV. The Prednisone infusion took all but an hour to coat my body. It ran its course causing me to become dazed and agitated as it passed through my system. It apparently worked because I was feeling relived of the fevers and chills.

My Second Hospital Stay

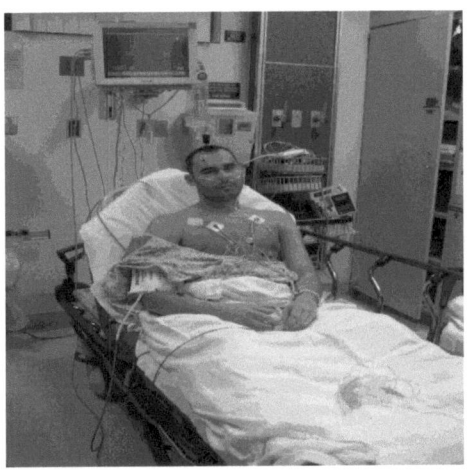

I was shivering so severe in bed; it was like I was in convolutions! Nicole woke up to see if I was okay. She got the thermometer and read it as 104.1 degrees. It had only been 2 days since I left the hospital.

I remember Nicole and myself waiting in the emergency room praying that God would have his mighty hand over our situation. As I spent the next three days in the hospital, I was administered different antibiotics.

I was also administered another high dose round of the Prednisone

(100 mg's). The 100 mg's was ordered to be administered over the next three days and the antibiotics for the next 10 days. In the hospital, I developed severe mouth sores. The doctors told me it was from the antibiotics I was on. They prescribed me something called Nystatin, a "swish and swallow." It was a yellowish, orange citrus tasting, thick concoction. It didn't seem to work!

Over the next few days my mouth sores turned into pits. I specifically remember 7 large pits. They were large enough for me to put the tip of my tongue into them! The ones on the inside of my cheeks felt like if I were to blow my cheeks up with air, my sides would leak air because my cheeks were so thin because the pits were so deep. The mouth sores that hurt the worst were the ones on the roof of my mouth. Needless to say, I lost weight due to not eating because of pain in my mouth. I have weighed 180 pounds ever since high school and I quickly dropped to 164 pounds in about a 2 week span.

The doctors continued to treat me for Pneumonia with antibiotics. The mouth sores still prevailed and chest x-rays were ordered to confirm the existence of Pneumonia. Because I was in the hospital, my kidney doctor and I were in contact every day. The doctor ordered another 24-hour urine analysis. This time when the results came back they yielded almost 5000 grams of protein! This is a huge number since a "normal" person, at the most, excretes about 150 g of protein in a 24-hour time frame. This alone, other than me not being able to breath and me feeling like crap, was a topic of huge concern. A serious conversation about me starting chemotherapy started to arise and this was a scary topic for both my wife and me.

Let me tell you about chemotherapy. Individuals on chemo have a reduction in fertility rather you are a female or male. My wife and I are a younger couple and it's our dream to have kids. We love kids! It was very discouraging to hear there was a possibly we wouldn't be able to have kids, if I opted for the chemotherapy treatment. Lupus patients who undergo chemotherapy treatment have an 80% remission rate. So we were contemplating my health or perusing our dreams. So do I take the chemotherapy treatment or do I not. More to come a little later!

My hopes and mindset changed one particular night while I was in the hospital. The majority of my family lives in the Central Valley (Fresno, Ca.) My immediate family and I are close. We speak on the phone once a day. Actually, for this particular hospital visit, my cell phone bill was over $600! (Nicole and I upped our plans shortly after receiving our bill.) I had been in contact with both of my sisters, Stephanie and Susan, earlier that day. They knew I was going to spend another night in the hospital and they decided to surprise me by driving 4.5 hours. It was about 6:00 pm, I was listening to the radio station (on the TV), playing solitary, when the door swung open. I saw these bright balloons and these shining individuals, which resembled my sisters. I had to honestly look twice because I didn't believe it was them! I just called Stephanie's house and her husband, Jeff, said that she was outside and she would call me back. Here they were walking into my hospital room! My eyes filled with tears, I couldn't believe it. It was so good to see them! They needed to see me and I needed to see them. We hung out for a few hours and they left for the night. The next morning they came back and kept me company, until it was time for them to go home. This was a great surprise for me. I remember telling family not to come to the hospital because I didn't want them to go out of their way for me. Little did I know it at the time, but I needed them there more then they or I knew. I honestly think my sisters presents lifted my spirit and helped me heal internally. With my wife by my side I rested the remainder of the day and continued to do what people do in the hospital, try and get out.

The next day my fever diminished, (as a side note, patients with Lupus generally runs at a lower temperature. My temperature is always around 96.7 degrees.) I wasn't feeling as bad and I was able to leave the hospital because I was "clinically stable." As I slipped my hospital shoes back on I took one last look into my room and wished to never see it again. Little did I know, I would have another go-around with my Lupus, the hospital and my shoes and I would soon be looking out the window wishing to get out once more.

My Third Hospital Stay

It had been about a month since my last encounter with my hospital slippers. I was feeling better and my energy level was on the rise. I did notice, however, that I was having a difficult time catching my breath after long conversations. I also noticed that catching my breath got more difficult as I performed the same daily tasks. I remember a time getting the mail and walking back up stairs. Just from climbing 14 stairs, my finger nails and toes turned blue. I was gasping for air! This gasping and blueness lasted for about 2 minutes and I would return back to "normal." *(What's normal for me at this point?)*

The next couple of days resulted in the same characteristics: Shortness of breath, blue finger and toe nails, and me starting to cough up blood! At first I didn't think too much about coughing up the blood, besides it was only about a quarter of a spoon full. After one day of constant coughing up of blood, SOB (shortness of breath), and blue extremities, I determined it was time to call the doctor. I explained to her the situation and she wanted me to get x-rays. This was on a Friday. The doctor arranged for x-rays, I had them taken and went home. I wasn't feeling too bad and my wife and I made plans to go surfing the next morning, if I was feeling up to it.

The next morning we woke up, took our Saturday morning walk on the beach with our coffee, and decided we were up to the challenge of going surfing. As we were both struggling to stretch on our wetsuits, I noticed that my cell phone was off. I guess my batteries had run dead. I plugged my phone in and turned it on. As we were heading out the door, I noticed a new message on my cell. I listened to it. The message revealed some interesting news! According to my doctor, the x-rays determined I had Pneumonia and that I needed to check myself into the hospital ASAP. Nicole, overseeing my face asked who left the message. I told her that you aren't going to like this message and that I needed to go check myself into the hospital.

There we were, in our wetsuits, surfboards in-hand. I replayed the Dr's message out loud for the both of us to hear. Nicole response was, "You have got to be kidding me!" I felt good enough to go surfing and was so discouraged I was going to have to go back to the hospital. We had a quick discussion of not to go surfing and to take the request serious. I changed, Nicole packed my play bag (which consisted of various things to do like: books to read, my bible, binoculars, headphones and writing material) and discouragingly, I was ready to put on my hospital shoes.

Based on the last few hospital stays, I was very disappointed because I was fully aware that I was going to spend a couple of days in the hospital. I was, by no means, getting use to the hospital stays and like most people staying in the hospital, was longing for the day I got to break out, even before I went in. I was dragging my feet as I gathered myself. I wanted to wake up from the nightmare I knew I was heading into. I knew from experience this was going to be miserable. I wanted nothing more to do then not to go into the hospital. As I slowly got ready to leave, I remembered my school's basketball team was playing at a local high school. (I was the basketball coach for our school and most of the schools players are on the same travel team.) I decided to get a coffee and watch them play their game before I checked into the hospital. I wanted to get some enjoyment out of the beautiful day!

After watching the boys play, I made my way to the emergency room. Following the review of my records, the emergency doctor administered the first of 3 doses of Prednisone, monitored me for a while and assigned me to my hospital room. The room they put me in was like a dungeon, as I remember it. It was what the nurses called an "over flow" room. This room was an old operating room converted into a patient's room. The lights were intensely bright circles that beamed down like spot lights. When I opened the one and only window shade, I saw grey cold concrete. I was bummed to be in the dungeon. After one day of being in the dungeon, I asked (okay demanded) to be transferred to a different room. I knew there were better rooms then the one I was currently in. I was just in a great room a month ago! I told them that I can't start to heal physically until I can start to heal mentally. The nurses took my plea seriously and I scored the best room in the hospital!

This room had it all: ocean view from my hospital bed, a couch that folded out into a bed, a lounge chair and best of all a chair that rocked! This is all great for the outward feeling, but the fact was that I was in the hospital because I was sick and this Lupus thing was affecting not only my joints and kidneys, but now my lungs!

The doctors agreed chemotherapy and Prednisone was the best option for me at this point because of the way the immune disease was playing "hopscotch" with my internal organs. Nicole and I knew we probably were going to have to make this decision and discussed the options earlier. Chemotherapy is a serious drug. It kills all cells, good and bad. It can affect fertility in both females and males. We researched Lupus, the treatments for Lupus and the affects of the treatments. We knew the possibility of my fertility would be reduced, due to the chemotherapy. We saw a fertility doctor before hand and back in January and had my sperm frozen for future use, just in case. Though I am optimistic and pray that we can conceive naturally down the road, it was a wise decision to have those little swimmers on reserve because of the severity of my disease.

Though at the time I didn't tell my family about me starting the chemotherapy, they knew in my voice that there was more to what I was telling them. My sister's tried to make another surprise visit, but I caught them. Mad at the fact they were trying to love me and surprise me, (I'm telling you the medicine is worse than the disease sometimes), I asked them to turn around and go home. They agreed to do as I wished. After about an hour of thinking about them and the treatment I was about to go through with the chemotherapy, I called back crying and pleaded with them to come down. They agreed and I waited impatiently for their arrival. *At this point in time, I need my wife and family there for support and I knew it and they knew it. I got through the next couple of days because of their love, prayers and support.*

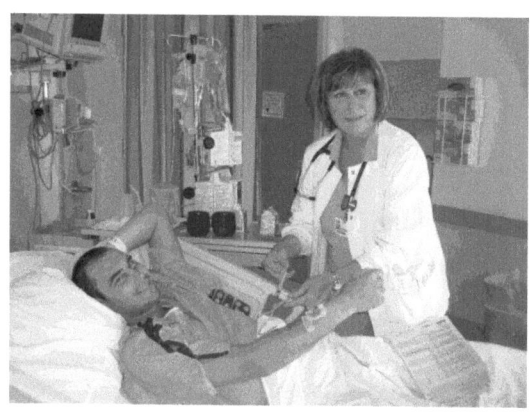

1ST CHEMOTHEREPY TREATMENT

I was scared! All I thought about was that I wanted to get better and that I wanted to have children, of our own (the natural way). I had this uncompromising view of each treatment of Chemotherapy I got induced with, the chances of Nicole and I having kids decreases. I was torn because of this, but was reassured because I had banked my swimmers knowing this situation might arise. Needless to say, this was still a hard decision for us and a decision those who come to it will have to make on their own. You will know what to do, just remember you want to be at your kids little league games, swim meets, cheerleading competitions and weddings. This treatment will get me there; this treatment will get you there.

The doctors said I should prepare for the side-effect from the chemotherapy. They said there was a possibility of nausea, balding, fatigue, and fertility loss. Thankfully, I didn't feel nausea, I already have thin hair (now I've got an excuse for it), and not sure about the fertility loss, yet.

BLOOD TRANSFUSION

Let's add another procedure to hospital visit 3. I was anemic and the doctors suggested a blood transfusion. My platelets were low and needed to be raised. After a successful procedure, I wasn't anemic; I was feeling better and ready to go home.

I was "clinically stable" to leave the hospital, according to the doctors. I packed up all my belongings, signed all my release paperwork and put on my hospital shoes. Not only was I ready to leave, but I never wanted to go back. *(No matter how awesome the food and water views were.)*

My Fourth Hospital Stay

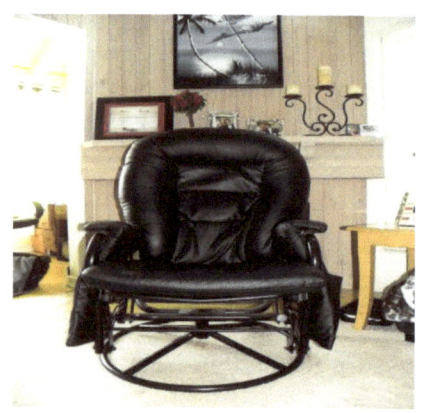

It's good to be going home! I have been in and out of the hospital for the last month. On this day, I was determined by the doctors to be "clinically stable" to leave. I sure don't want to go back. It was late afternoon by the time I was discharged from the hospital. The drive back to our house never looked so beautiful; ocean view all the way! For the next 10 minutes chatted with my wife, gazed at the sun glazing off the ocean ripples and smiled with optimistic joy because I was going home!

It was good to be home! I felt like a king rocking in my chair! There was nothing more I would rather be doing. After a great dinner, it was time for some much needed sleep. I took some sleeping meds and hit my pillow with heavy eyes. I woke up about 2:00 am to use the bathroom. As I swung my feet over the side of the bed, I noticed I felt very dizzy. As I stood up and made my way to the bathroom and almost fell over. I was starting to gasp for air! I couldn't breathe and my lungs hurting every time I took a breath! I was coughing too. I noticed a funny taste in my mouth. As I spit into the sink, I noticed it was red. As I focused my tired eyes they concluded that it was in fact blood! Wonderful, I thought, what else could possible go wrong with me. I was so excited to not be at the hospital. Now, with me gasping for air and coughing up blood, I was most definitely going to be wearing my hospital shoes again.

As I tried to breath, I woke my sleeping beauty up and explained to her the events that just happened. She asked if I was serious and quickly became convinced after she saw me grasping for air and after I showed her the blood I coughed up. Nicole shoved some clothes, cards and my bible into the duffle bag, which was packed with other items from the hospital visit just less than 12 hours ago, and we left *again* for the hospital.

Into the emergency room we went. I, again, recognized faces of doctors and nurses and they recognized me. One nurse in particular was trying to start my IV but wasn't successful securing a line. With the syringe in my arm, blood was pumping out of my arm getting all over me and the gurney! It was like in the movies where it squirts into the air every time the heart beats. Never had I an experience where I passed out, but I had a feeling I was about to experience it for the first time. As I became nauseous, I asked the nursing assistant for a container to throw-up in. I remember him handing me a small container. I told him that I needed something bigger. At this point I recall the doctors, nurses, and nursing assistants' voices getting softer. I also remember me floating above myself. I was able to see me, the doctors, nurses, assistants, Nicole and the top of the cabinet (which was dusty.) I wasn't scared, but rather calm and collect. I remember thinking that it was weird and interesting at the same time. My next recollection was of me hearing voices get louder and the nurse asking me to lie all the way down. After a while, I refocused and told the nurse that the top of the cabinet was dirty. I am 6'3 and the top of the cabinet was about 8 feet tall. This was the first time I've experienced anything like this and the doctor said it was called Autoscopy, which was an out of the body experience.

After the out of body experience, I was escorted to my hospital room. This time the blood I was spitting up was from Alveolar Hemorrhaging and I was induced with another round of high dose prednisone (100 mg's.) Interestingly, I have always weighed about 180 pounds, since high school. I lost weight, due to mouth sours, and three weeks ago weighed in at 164 pounds. At this point in time I was tipping the scales at 202 pounds! Again, the medications are sometimes worse than the disease. The Prednisone was causing me to retain large amounts of water and was increasing my hunger. The hunger increase was due to a signal in my brain not registering that I was full. With my mouth sores gone, I was eating everything in sight. The hospital food was surprisingly good. I usually went with the dinner choice of: choice steak, mashed potatoes, chicken fingers, (with barbeque sauce,) salad with lemon, 2 vanilla puddings, 2 vanilla ice creams, and water. *The high dose of Prednisone was not only causing me to retain water, but it increased my hunger as-well, no wonder I gained 38 pounds in 4 weeks!*

After three days in the hospital, I was fed-up, upset, ready to leave, but still had my game face on because I knew this is what it was going to take to get me better. One major aspect I was lacking was sleep. I know the doctors, nurses, nurse assistants and many others who came into my room throughout the day were trying to get me well, but one needs sleep. I was curious on how many visits I received throughout one day so I decided to journal them. Here are the times:

Day 1 AM	Day 2 PM
6:00 am Blood work	12:00 pm Lunch time
6:10 am MRI on knee	12:20 pm Pulmonary Dr. visit
7:00 am Glucose test	2:00 pm Vital sign check
7:10 am Vital sign check	2:10 pm Nurse check-up
8:00 am Nebulizer treatment (for my lungs)	5:00 pm Dinner
8:15 am Meds	5:30 pm Glucose check
8:15 am Breakfast (I didn't mind this interruption)	5:40 pm Vital sign check
9:00 am Overseeing Dr. hospital check-up	6:00 pm Insulin given
10:00 am Rheumatologist Dr. check-up	7:00 pm Vital sign check
10:20 am Steroid infusion	7:30 pm Meds
11:00 am Glucose test	9:00 pm Vital sign check
11:30 am Vital sign check	11:00 pm Vital sign check
11:35 am Kidney Dr. check-up	11:10 pm Blood drawn
	1:00 am More blood work
	2:00 am Vital sign check

That's it! Just 28 different times where I was checked, woken up, or was stabbed with a needle! Like I said before, people in the hospital are in there to get better, but rest sure sounded great at anytime of the day.

While in the hospital, my mom and sister Susan made a trip from the Central Valley to see me. They needed to see me for themselves to confirm that I was alright. They were there to comfort and calm me. I was glad to see them and they were relieved to see me. Again, Lupus is an interesting disease. At this point in time, I looked far better then I felt. Metaphorically, compared to a 1967 Mustang my sister Susan use to own; the car looked awesome, beautiful, shiny, it even looked fast and flawless; but it ran like a pony on crutches, it was not reliable and would leave you stranded 9 out of 10 times. I am glad my family was there to assist with my emotional needs. I was tired, cranky and was eager to go home. I needed them to lean on and that's just what they let me do.

After the third day, I was clinically cleared to be discharged from the hospital. I packed up all my belongings, put on my hospital shoes, and was wheeled out of my room. My mom drove me home in my truck which, had been at the hospital for a week now. I prayed this would be the end of my hospital days for awhile. I mean really who needed to be at home in February anyway.

My Next Hospital Visit

I don't know when the next hospital visit will be. I pray I will not have another incident which will put me back into my hospital shoes. I have read on websites that a typical Lupus patient will be admitted to the hospital 7 days per year. *I would like to know how they determined who a typical Lupus patient is!* I would like for the treatments to put my Lupus into remission. I would like to get back to my old self again. *Or would I?*

This experience has opened doors for me. It has allowed me to view life differently. I never wish *not* to have gotten this disease. I have it for a reason. I believe, I will have Lupus for the rest of my life or until we find a cure for it and as far as my health in the future, only time will tell. This is just one of many obstacles, bumps, valleys, triumphs, joys and fears thus far in my young life. I am a fighter and I will fight this until the end. My battle for now is Lupus.

CHAPTER 6
MY MEDS

Growing up I never took any sort of medication. Well okay, I was never really sick like I am now but, if I had a headache for instance I would drink some coffee. If I sprained my ankle I would ice it. That's it! I'm 28 years old and up to this point never influenced my body with any medications, painkillers or substances that caused my body to react the way it is currently reacting. I'm not good at naming all my medications. However, I did take organic chemistry in college and was able to identify chemicals using nomenclature names. The list I am about to share with you is long. I just wanted for whoever is reading this to have a list to compare, in case they are going through the same treatments as me or for those who would like to know what to expect. (Please see next page.)

My Medicine Intake
Date Started January 2009
As of 01-26-2010

Ativan (Lorazepam 0.5 mg)	Levaquin 500 mg
Ativan (Lorazepam 1 mg)	Lidocaine 2% Viscous Solution
Atrovent HFA Inhaler	Lisinopril 10 mg
Calcium 500 mg	Norvasc (Amlodipine Besylate 5 mg)
Cefuroxime Axetil 500 mg	Nystatin 100,000 Units/ml s
Cellcept 500 mg	One A Day
Cytoxin (Cyclophosphamide mg IV injection)	Plaquenil (Hydrooxychloroquine 200 Mg)
Darvocet-N 100 (Propoxyphen-APAP 100-650 mg)	Potassium CL 20 MEQ
Diflucan (Fluconazole 100 mg)	Prednisone 100 Mg, 60 Mg, 50 Mg exc..
Dilaudid (Hydromorpone 2 mg)	Prevacid 30 Mg
Diovan 160 mg	Proair HFA 90 MCG Inhaler
Diovan 320 Mg	Prochlorperazine 10 mg
Etodolac 400 mg	Triamcinolone 0.1% Paste
Folic Acid 1 Mg	Ultram ER 200 Mg
Furosemide 20 mg	Vicodin (Hydrocodone-APAP 5-500)
Insulin IV	Zaleplon 10 mg

The above list is medication I have taken since my diagnosis of Lupus. Of all the medication I am on or was on, Prednisone was the most challenging. I was on 60 mg's of prednisone for 3 months! In the hospital the Prednisone was increased to 100 mg's over 3 separate treatments, each time I was there! According to the doctors the major side effects of this medication include: Severe allergic reactions (rash; hives; itching; difficulty breathing; tightness in the chest; swelling of the mouth, face, lips, or tongue); appetite loss; black tarry stools; changes in menstrual periods (I didn't have this one); convulsions; depression; diarrhea; dizziness; exaggerated sense of well-being; fever; general body discomfort; headache; increased pressure in the eye; joint or muscle pain; mood swings (big time for me); muscle weakness (I experienced this one); personality changes; prolonged sore throat, cold, or fever; puffing of the face (AKA moon face and I had it); severe nausea or vomiting; swelling of feet or legs; unusual weight gain (yep); vomiting material that looks like coffee grounds; weakness; weight loss, difficulty sleeping (I had this one); feeling of a whirling motion; increased appetite; increased sweating (yes); indigestion; mood changes; nervousness. My specific side effects were mainly: Puffiness in the face; joint pain in the knees (that's why I had an X-ray and MRI on my knees and the crutches); acne; mouth sores; severe agitation or mood swings; shortness of breath, increased appetite; night sweats; and difficulty sleeping. *(Even with taking sleeping medications.)*

Let me tell you about a side effect called moon face. It's is where ones face gets extremely fat or puffy in the face due to water retention from Prednisone. To me, when I looked in the mirror, my face didn't look like my face. When online, I read about many people who were on Prednisone and felt the same way because of the moon face. I had students ask me why my face was getting fatter. (Remember I taught at the middle school level and sometimes there not the nicest of people.) I told them that sometimes when the weather gets hot my face expands. (Because of the diagnosis being so new to me, neither they nor my staff knew about my diagnosis or what I was going through at the time.) It was challenging up to this point to say the least, but I knew taking the medications it was necessary for the time being. For my sisters Stephanie and Susan, all I can say is "Hey, hey, hey"

My lab results have been looking better after the first round of chemotherapy. I got news from my kidney doctor that I didn't have to see him for 3 months. My last 24-hour urine test was at 376 mg's of protein and no traces of blood. My lungs still hurt and the lung doctor said it was from the inflammation around the lungs called pleurisy. This, according to the doctor is a result from Lupus itself (called Lupus Lung) and once we put the Lupus into remission, the lungs should not hurt anymore.

As of May 1, 2009 I was down to 20 mg of prednisone. I have been feeling better and we will see how much better I feel after my second round of chemotherapy. It is scheduled for May 9th 2009. The doctor is also testing my anemia. For this test I get to poop in a bag and the lab gets to analyze the results.

SECOND CHEMO TREATMENT

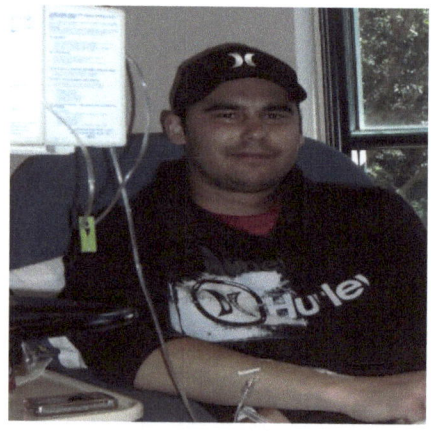

The second round of chemotherapy was scheduled for Saturday May 9th 2009. However, due to paperwork error the procedure couldn't take place. This was difficult for me because I prepared mentally and physically for the treatment. Needless to say, I was upset, but it was rescheduled for the following Wednesday.

Wednesday came too fast! The pre-register nurse told me that the procedure would take 6 hours. I didn't remember the first treatment taking that long. I was explaining the amount time and procedure to my sister Stephanie and she asked me if I remembered playing Candy Land throughout the last treatment in the hospital. I didn't remember, probably due to the high dose of medications I was on. She tried her best to jar my memory and asked me if I remembered "the drinking game." Stephanie was told by the nurse to make sure I drank lots of fluids throughout the chemotherapy procedure. Each turn I had while playing Candy Land, I was made to drink water. It sounded fun to me, sure wish I remembered it.

I didn't get nauseous during the treatment. The doctor ordered me anti-nauseous medication and the round of chemotherapy. I was super tired after the treatment, and this was probably due to me being anemic. I worked the following days and longed for the weekend.

That Friday when I got home from work I went to bed at 6:00pm. Only waking up a few times to use the bathroom, I woke up the next morning at 7:00 am. That Saturday, I met up with some friends to go surfing. I ended up surfing (more like paddling due to lack of waves) for about three hours. I had fun but had to take many breaks because it was difficult to breath due to the Lupus Lung.

May 27th, 2009
Tired

It was a Wednesday, 2 weeks after my last chemotherapy treatment. I felt tired. I was tired when I woke up, tired as I took each step throughout the day, tired as I responded to the 'Hi, how are you today's?" Tired as I slurped up my Chinese food noodles for lunch, tired as I drank water from my bottle, tired as I drove home and thought about my pillow, tired as I slipped my shoes off before I came into the house, tired as I used the bathroom, tired as I gave my wife a hug, and tired as I climbed into bed for a long nap. This wasn't a normal feeling for me. I was sure it was from the chemotherapy. The exhaustion lasted about 4 days and my energy level started to pick up again, yet not as it was in November 2008.

Though the exhausting days were very heavy for me, there was some enlightening news. My Rheumy doctor called me and said I could start Cellcept. She said that my blood levels looked normal enough and she felt comfortable to have me stop the chemotherapy and start this other, less potent, immunosuppressant. I wanted to peruse this option because I was clinically looking better and wanted not to be on the Cytoxin, (chemotherapy.)

Cellcept was discussed as an alternative to chemotherapy because it wouldn't cause the destruction to my fertilization as the chemotherapy was. I was on 500 mg a day and I was to increase it to 1000 mg per day after the first 10 days.

May 29th 2009
What Hairy Back?

I have been reducing my steroid, Prednisone, for the last 5 weeks. I was directed by my doctor to decrease 10 mg's per week until I reached 10 mg's. I was finally taking just 10 mg's and my face diminished from balloon size to more of a football size. I was looking more and more like myself and feeling more like myself as well.

One side effect, not only as I researched but experienced, was that Prednisone allowed individuals taking the medication to experience hair growth. My hair growth congregated on my back. (Too bad it wasn't on my head!) I have always had a hairless, sexy, and flawless back. *(Okay, I have all mentioned above except the last two.)* It was difficult for me to have hair accumulating on my back; I didn't want to be always looking in the mirror at my hairy back because of the reflection of the person looking back. (Do to the prednisone; he looked like a person who was afraid of losing his lunchtime snack so he stuffed it into his cheeks like a hamster.) The indication of the hair growth on my back came to me as I was standing outside with my shirt off in the wind. Like streamers on a child's bike, I could feel the wind, ever so gently, whirl my newly acquainted back hairs. It was time to bring my sexy back!

My wife and I went to the store and picked up some hair removal for men. It was a spray, leave on for 10 minutes and wipe off application. Skeptical of the unlikelihood it was actually that easy, we followed the procedures and to our excitement it worked. Ha! No more tickling of the wind as I am getting the mail. My flawless back was rejuvenated!

Not only was my back shiny, soft, and hair free, but my legs now too. I have always had hairy legs and the chemotherapy was causing the hair on my legs to fall out in patches. My legs looked like a battleship board with hit-and-miss patches of missing hair. I took care of that problem with my hair trimmer. I set it to the lowest setting and gave the old legs a buzz cut. I just thought of it as tapering, as runners do. After the hair was buzzed off, I cut 3 seconds off my mile time. I now can run it in under 15 minutes☺

June 11, 2009
My Pee and Me!

Today I am carrying my 24-hour pee apparatus. It's not the most pleasant way of going through my day, but it's one of the best tests to determine if I have protein being excreted from my kidney. This will allow us to know if the chemotherapy is working on the kidneys.

There is a staff room in the back of my classroom and there a refrigerator is found tucked into the corner. My urine needs to be kept cold at all times. I know that my colleagues are curious to why I keep going in and out of the refrigerator with a gym bag. I haven't revealed to them that I needed to have my urine saved for protein analysis; I didn't think they needed to know.

I am continuing to drop 1 mg of Prednisone each week. I am now currently at 8 mgs. I do feel some side effects of coming off the Prednisone. I am sluggish, very fatigued, and still have a fat face. The nausea I feel is probably from the 1000 mg of Cellcept I am taking. Each day is a new day for me. I'm looking forward to the summer, as school is out in one week!

July 4, 2009
Fireworks and Family

My sister Stephanie, her husband Jeff, two daughters Jillian and Kayden spent the 4th of July with us. They visited for about a week and we had a blast. We went to Disneyland, the aquarium, the swap meet and hung out on the beach. My sister Susan was also down for the 4th and stayed at a nearby location because 6 people in a one bedroom condo is very challenging especially with a 2 and a half year old and a 7 month old, just starting to speed crawl.

My sister Stephanie's favorite day is the 4th of July. She has always been in awe, like most of us, of the spectacular firework shows. This is the 3rd consecutive year Stephanie and her family has spent the holiday with us. This year's extravaganza was no exception.

Our 4th of July ritual begins with us waking up, eating breakfast and spending the rest of our time together on the beach. Jeff always spends too much of his time setting up his canopy while the rest of us find ways to permanently attach amounts of sand into our hair, teeth and pockets. We usually break for lunch, as we walk back up to the condo and devour sandwiches. (This year it was pastrami.) We then make our way back to the surf and sand. I however, dealing with my extreme fatigue, needed a nap. So the baby and I shut our eyes as the rest were claiming to the sand once more.

Dinner time came too soon and we found ourselves around the grill enjoying hamburgers. With nightfall, our oversized blanket awaited my family. From our spot on the beach we could see the firework shows from Huntington Beach, Long Beach, Palos Verde and the Los Alamitos Naval station. The lights were a spectacular venue but what made it even more special was that the night was shared with my family.

Along with all the activities we embarked on, one of the best moments for me was surfing with my sister Stephanie. We went out on a sunny afternoon and the waves were perfect. She amazed me as she would stand over and over again. Good thing we captured her perfection on camera because nobody would have believed us.

My family's stay with Nicole and I was fantastic and although, I did feel bad throughout their visit because I had to take necessary naps. There were times where I was just exhausted. Naps I am learning are an essential part of this recovery process. People recover in their sleep and if you are not sleeping then you are recovering very slowly. I am trying to understand this process and taking napping and sleeping very serious. For those going though this crucial time in their process, remember to listen to what your body is telling you. If you need sleep, get it!

July 9, 2009
Teaching in the Summer

I am down to 4 mg's of Prednisone. I am currently taking 1000 mg's of Cellcept, Diovan for blood pressure, one-a-day (vitamins), 1 mg of Folic Acid, 500 mg's of Plaquinell, and 1000 mg's of vitamin D. I definitely feel the remnants of lowering my Prednisone. My elbow joints, specifically, are reminding me of the reduction of the steroid in my system. The pain is temporary; as it only lasts up to 4 days after my reduction then the pain diminishes. My face is almost back to normal and my protein is holding at 234 g's.

This year I am teaching summer school. It is from 8-12 for 5 weeks. All of my kids are in the 6th grade and taking the class because they failed it the first time they tried. I take it upon myself to dedicate as much effort and as much instruction as possible to clearly educate these students in the area of math. Thus far, half way through the summer school session, they have shown much improvement and the efforts I am putting in feels successful.

Day after day I am forced to acknowledge how fatigued I am. My daily routine consists of me: waking up, taking my meds, eating breakfast, teaching at summer school, eating lunch, taking a nap, hanging out with my wife, playing a little, eating dinner, taking more meds and then going to bed. That's it in a nut shell. This seems pretty normal in my eyes, except for the fatigue, naps and the consumption of medication. I am content up to this point because I know the journey I have gone through has helped me get to where I am at.

July 17, 2009
Coughing and Spitting up Green Stuff

For the past three days I have noticed a "tingle" in my throat. Today I coughed up green mucus. Not good since Nicole and I were to leave to Cayucos Beach. I have to take it serious whenever I feel ill because the medications I take lower my immune system. Currently, I am taking Cellcept and Prednisone. I called the doctor, explained the symptoms and explained my travel plans. The doctor made time to see me today at 2 pm. After he prescribed me antibiotics, we hit the road to the beach.

July 22, 2009
Getting Better

I was prescribed antibiotics and have been taking them for the last 5 days. I am starting to feel better and coughing up less green mucus. I also got some test results back from blood work and a 24-hr urine test I had done last week. They were the best results since I was diagnosed with Lupus! My kidney secretion of protein was at 192 mg's. (150 mg's is considered "normal") I am very thankful and pray for continued improvement.

August - December 2009
Stronger

I am getting stronger, I am taking less medication and my labs are looking great!

January 26, 2010
My Pee and Me

I carried around my pee again for a full day. I am starting to get good at disguising it from my coworkers, though some know about my condition and why I have to do it. The urinalysis on the 24-hour urine came back at 172 mg's of protein excretion. The normal range is up to 150 mg's of protein excretion. It has been dropping the last couple of months.

My blood work is also looking good, with the exception of my double strand DNA which is at 124. The ranges are 0-4 (normal) 5-10 (look at labs) and greater than 10 which means there is a response in the immune system. The dsDNA and the protein excretion are the main items used for tracking and maintaining my Lupus.

February 14, 2010
Valentine's Day In The Hospital

I will always remember February 14, 2009. It was a Valentine's Day I'll never forget because I was in the hospital. Not too romantic, though Nicole tried! This year was spent with my wife and family. My sister Stephanie, Susan, niece Jillian and Kayden spent the weekend with us. The weather was perfect (70 ish) and we had a blast just hanging out on the beach, enjoying each other's company. I kept catching myself thinking that

I am so glad and fortunate I am here now when compared to last year at this time. Thank you, thank you, and thank you!

CHAPTER 7
LIVING WITH LUPUS

LIFE ALTERING

Lupus is a life-altering disease. For me it has changed my daily walk (*literally and figuratively.*) I have gone to a doctor's office once each and every week since being diagnosed with Lupus, for about the first 3-4 months. This has allowed me to have a different perspective and view the world differently. I have a different spin on life. I hear people complain, but what they are complaining about doesn't seem too essential to me. (*I don't want to be a hypocrite because looking back on my days; I too would be the complainer in the wind.*) I overheard one person complaining about how their legs hurt when they get up in the morning. I wanted to ask them if they knew what it was like for their legs to hurt so hard, it was impossible to walk. That's the hurt I felt some days. Through all the pain and complaining I did do, I knew there are still people around me in worse shape or having a worse day then what I am having. I don't want to pretend and say everything is fine, when in fact it's not. I don't want to cover up for those who are in my situation and in pain. I don't want people to think that Lupus is a mild sickness the acquirer has. I don't want to down play the disease either. There are some Lupus patients who need to be cautious of the sun and there are some Lupus patients that need to be cautious of stairs because they can't walk up them. Lupus patients and people come in different varieties, some are more ripe then others and some need to be left on the vine for more ripening. Living with Lupus has allowed me to have this perspective. I know I am fortunate because I have God and my family behind me and that is more than many others have. I know I have this disease for a reason. I feel, I need to get my story out to family, friends, husbands, wife's, uncles, aunts, sisters, brothers and others who have Lupus and are facing challenging times in their lives. As I researched men with Lupus, I found it difficult to find information on men with symptoms similar to mine. Hopefully, this book will help others who are going through situations like mine.

PEOPLES OPINIONS

While doing research on Lupus, I e-mailed and have had conversations with many who have Lupus. Most are women which have a wide range of Lupus like symptoms and most I've spoken to have the skin rash or joint pain. I guess I'm the one who drew the cards which states I have the joint pain, kidney issues and lung issues. That's okay! Like I said before I have this for a reason. I have Lupus, Lupus doesn't have me!

Because of the medication due to my Lupus, I have heard comments flow from people's mouths. For example, other than me looking like a balloon head, with aches who limps, I look normal. I don't feel normal, yet. Again, I'm like my sisters beautiful, poor and not running so good Mustang. I have a temporary handicap pass. When I step out of my truck and take a few limps, I feel as though people are looking at me thinking "Why is this young man illegally parking in handicap." I had an old man go as far as calling me a phony. (*I don't park in handicap when my knees are working correctly.*) I just remember I am doing the best job I can with this disease and all I can do is take one day at a time. Sometimes I need to break those days up into morning, afternoon and night. Even then I need to break it up into individual hours, but it's manageable and I am making it.

NEW ADVENTURES

I haven't been able to run up and down the basketball court as I used to. I haven't been able surf as much due to my chemotherapy and my immune system being suppressed. I haven't been able to run in races my wife and I used to run in. There are many things I haven't done since I have been diagnosed with Lupus. However, there are many other activities I am doing because of my disease!

It's challenging, but I think of having Lupus like going on an adventure. I think of other activities I can do. I read more, play easier, live slower, and enjoy my surrounding more, I like to fish and love photography now. I would view these activities differently if it hadn't been for my diagnosis. Though I'm still figuring it all out, I am content with my new lifestyle. I have only had Lupus for 12 months, up to this point in the story, and I am optimistic that someday I probably will be able to dunk a basketball again, hit the 400 foot home runs and keep up with my wife in a 5k race. Until then my eyes are open, my ears listening and my heart content on life. I am learning to relax. I am figuring out that sometimes the only person who can allow for you to relax is yourself. I am trying to allow for that to happen….. Yea, I'm relaxing for a while.

CHAPTER 8

BE CAREFULE FOR WHAT YOU WISH FOR

I remember praying for people who were sick and asking God to take the sickness from them and put it into me. I always thought I could handle it better because I was strong. One day my sister was in a boating accident. The boats' propeller cut her leg as she climbed onto the boat from the water. The propeller ripped out her fibula as she was sucked under the boat. After the engine was turned off, you could hear her under the boat as she hit the bottom of it. As she was pulled up, the realization of what occurred hit home. Shear panic broke out! Blood everywhere! Bone missing! 15 by 6 inch gash in her leg! Just as this was happening another boater, who happened to be a surgeon specializing in trauma, was fishing on his day off was passing by. He climbed aboard and knew exactly what artery in her leg to clamp to prevent her from bleeding to death. That day Stephanie almost died at the lake. I recall praying to God that I should have been the one who was injured. Over the last weeks, I too, could not walk, as was the case with my sister Stephanie during the months after her accident. Though I didn't have a bone ripped from my leg, though it honestly felt like there was. The pain was excruciating! Just so you know, today my sister can run, walk, kick really hard, *(I know from experience as she has literally kicked me in the back side many times)* and functions normally without a limp. She has gotten through her incident just as I am going to get through mine. She is and will continue to be my inspiration!

Other times I have prayed for people including times when family members were feeling ill like: when my grandmother had cancer and was going through her treatments, my grandfather who had a stint and hernias, my wife's grandfather who also had a stint and major complications from it and my sister Susan who was sick with God only knows what. I would ask God to take their sickness from them and to put it into me. I always thought I could handle it better than them and I would rather be the one sick than them. I would be willing to carry it on my back and I would be willing to bear the burden for them. I was optimistic that if I were to have their illness, I would conquer it and move on with my life. Now Lupus presents itself and to those questions raised above; we shall see, we shall see how I do handling the disease!

Though I am not angry, I do find it interesting, I now have a sickness I can't get rid of. Lupus will always affect me. I know I can handle this, but only with God, my wife and my family by my side. It's not only me who is being affected by Lupus it's those around me, my entire family. I know they are with me every step of the way and together we can accomplish anything. I am grateful for their love, support and comfort.

CHAPTER 9

MY LEGACY

Can you be too young to know what your legacy should be? When my time comes, I know how I would like to be remembered. I would like to be remembered as a man who: loved the Lord, a man who loved his wife and family, a man who loved his kids, a man who made a positive influence on people around him, a man who gave more then he took and a man who honestly tried to help and educate others with Lupus. These are all notions I would like to be remembered as.

I haven't fulfilled my purpose, yet. However, knowing what I would like to accomplish helps direct me in to where I need to go. I do understand fulfilling my legacy is going to take work and much effort along the way. I have a saying which goes like this, "If you want to go somewhere fast, go alone. If you want to go somewhere far, take others." My family and friends have been battling Lupus with me from the beginning. They will be with me for the long haul. They are my others! We will fight until the end.

So to answer the question of can you be too young to know what your legacy should be is no. I have an idea, passion and vision of how I can make a difference on this earth. I know how I would like to be remembered. I just need to accomplish the goals at-hand.

CHAPTER 10

MY LOVE

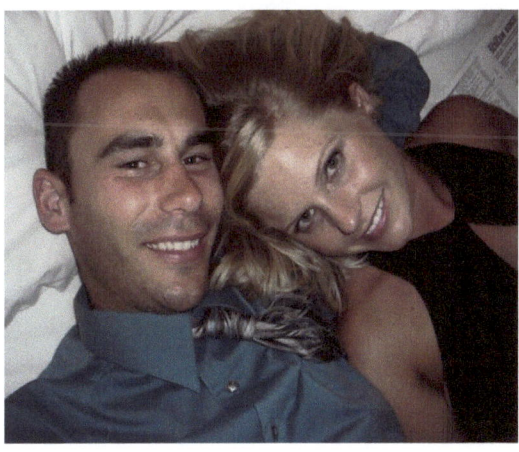

My love, my joy, and my sunshine! I would, without a second thought, lay my life down for my love, Nicole. I often wonder how I became such a lucky man and how I was able to marry such an amazing girl. She truly is my very own angel! She has been my rock in many times of need. Three years ago we got married. That was the second best day in my life. The first was accepting Jesus Christ into my life. Nicole being 5'3 and me towering over her at 6'3, I want nothing more than to hold her over my head as high as I can for all to see her. To let the readers know a little more about her, she is just as beautiful on the inside as the outside!

I know I'm in love because I feel it. I know I'm in love because I think it. I know I'm in love because when I'm enjoying the most beautiful things in life like: an amazing sunset, sunrise, the perfect wave, or dolphins performing acrobatic tricks for me; it's not perfect because my love is not by my side. I don't want to sound conceded but thankful because I could have captured many other girls' hearts, yet I am drawn to Nicole. The way her hand fits perfectly into mine, the taste of her lips, the kindness of her eyes and the sweetness of her touch fills every angle of my heart. I thank the Lord and Nicole every day for her and her love. It's so awesome to know that the person staring back at you loves you as much as you love them.

At the time I was diagnosed, in the hospital and going through chemotherapy treatments, my love was in nursing school. Nursing school is tuff enough by itself, let alone caring for someone who was very needy at times. I am so proud of her and have learned many characteristics from her. My bride is a great example of someone who gives more then she takes. She is always sacrificing things she likes and places she wants to go because of my wants or needs. She leads by example of putting others first.

Our first three years of marriage have been exciting. We moved away from our upbringing environments, our family was no longer a 10 minute drive away and we started new careers. Yes, life as we knew it was going as planned, but sometimes life doesn't go how *we* want for it to go.

The Lupus and treatments have been difficult. The chemotherapy throws a big conundrum into our future plans. We both love kids and it was one of our many serious conversations as we were dating. I love my wife and I want to be able to conceive kids with her. When you hear the words of "things happen for a reason" it doesn't hit home until those "things or events" are happening to you. It's time for us to take our stand and be firm in our faith with the Lord. I guess time will tell!

I look forward to many more happy years ahead of us. I look

forward to growing old with her. The medical happenings are unfortunate, but I have never blamed anyone for what I have or what I'm going through. Like I stated before, "I have Lupus for a reason." What doesn't break us makes us stronger. We are growing as a couple. We are stronger than before because our base is of our faith in our Lord. Everything else will fall into place. Yes, it is I who has Lupus, but it is we who are fighting the battle. Together we shall go on.

CHAPTER 11

MY FAITH

It's intriguing that when life is going good, we tend not to rely on God as much as we do when life is not going so well. I became a Christian in 2000. I have had my ups and down as a Christian. During my difficult times, I relied on God to get me through the tuff times. I prayed to Him with an honest heart. I read his word constantly and would seek him all times of the day. At times when I was getting 2 hours of sleep at night, (this lasted for about 8 weeks,) and I was with Him and He was with me. At times when I was getting stabbed with needles, I was seeking him. At times when I was in MRI machines, I would call on his name. All the times I was calling His name, he was there listening, answering and comforting me.

I know God doesn't give us more then we can handle. I have Lupus for a reason. I prayed I would have an open heart, a listening ear, and that my sight fixed on Him. I knew I had to do something more then to let Lupus run my life. I needed to take the position of, "I have Lupus, Lupus doesn't have me." I was and will continue to be my own advocate. I prayed for the doctors treating me. I prayed for God to give them the knowledge they needed to make a positive influence on their caring treatments. I prayed they would not treat me like a "cookie cutter patient." Again, this is where they only treat patients according to the textbook and according to the textbook; Lupus patients were woman, with joint pain, who had little internal complications, according to *some* doctors.

As I read, contemplated and meditated over the bible, I found some verses I would like to share. They are: Psalm 91 and 32 (also a favorite of my grandmother and grandfather, Verna and George respectively,) Psalm 37, Exodus 15:26, Mathew 21:22 and Job 5:18 just to name a few. The verses talk of being in the shadows of the Lords wing, trusting in Him, waiting for Him patiently, healing us, and for us to believe and receive in His name.

My friends no matter what situations, circumstances, problems or challenges I am facing I know there is someone out there in the world far worse then I. Someone who needs more help than me. We are only as strong as the Lord allows us to be. With him all things are possible, even the continuous battle with Lupus. It's because of Him, I am getting through this. My mom and I were talking the other day and she was telling me how all people's sickness is going to be no more in heaven. How I won't have to worry about Lupus in heaven, how many of you reading this with Lupus will not have this striking disease once the Lord comes. Until then, I will have my hospital shoes ready and do as Psalm 37:7 says, "Be still before the Lord and wait patiently for Him." With the bible as my playbook, the Lord, my wife, family and friends by my side I find strength, comfort and a drive to not only help myself, but to help and encourage others around me.

I've always believed there was power in prayer. Many times I have prayed for a person over a certain situation. Over the last few months, I know there have been many people praying for me. I have had friends pray for me at their small groups, in congregations as groups, by themselves and with me in person. I have prayed with my wife, friends and family. I am a witness of power in prayer! I have felt God's presents in my life, spiritually and physically!

One particular day, my mother and I were talking on the phone. I remember having a temperature of about 101 degrees, pressure in my head and my eyes burning. After we were done speaking to each other, I remember my mom praying for the listed symptoms above. I honestly kid you not, after she was finished praying for me, felt the pressure in my head fading away, my eyes burned less and less with each passing moment until they didn't burn and I felt the burning fever lift off me. All this occurred really fast, just after my mom finished praying for me. As my eyes watered from happiness, I could barely explain to my mom why I was weeping so hard. Power in pray is *really* powerful, I felt it for myself!

Why was I chosen to have this disease? My wife and I didn't expect this type of challenge in our lives. How are we going to get through this? What does this mean for our future? These are all questions pondered by the both of us. I love my wife and I would never wish for this situation. Fact of the matter is, I don't know why I was chosen to have this disease, but I do know I can make a positive difference because of it. My wife and I are going to get through this together, with the guidance from God. We have grown already in the short amount of time as a wedded couple and as a couple, of which one has an auto immune disease. Our future is in God's hands. Honestly, it's scary because we don't know what tomorrow brings. Sometimes I think it would be nice to know what the next day brings, but I also love living optimistically and enjoy walking with my faith. It's okay for us not to know what the future holds. As long as we have our trust in the Lord, we will be provided for.

CHAPTER 12

FUTURE OUTLOOK FOR LUPUP PATIENTS

A great online tool I use is called Lupus Foundation of America. (http://www.lupus.org) They have up to date information, message boards, information on local resources, and much more. I found myself on the discussion boards many times at night and early in the morning, when sleep was so far from me. I felt comfort knowing I can research and share information with others who have Lupus.

There is no cure for Lupus. However, with sciences techniques and medicines patients are living longer than before. The Lupus foundation of America states that "Patients with non-organ threatening aspects can look forward to a normal life span." Hum, what about the patients who are like me and have the organ threatening type of Lupus?

I'm not going to lie! It's great to surf the internet and see "new treatments" or alternative treatments for chemotherapy being discussed. However, when one such as myself, are going through the situation being discussed; the "new treatments" aren't always discussed in the office by the doctors. Pretty much, the treatment for my particular case is the same treatment that was preformed 40 years ago. Treat the kidney, lungs, and joints with chemotherapy (Cytoxin) and prednisone seem to be the norm. Not, saying that my doctors are misguiding me, but they seem to go by the textbooks no matter what age or race one is. If it had success before it probably will have success again, seems to be their take on my treatment. I got the impression that the treatment for Lupus patients fell into the "cookie cutter category." That is, for the doctors to follow the same protocol for all patients, when in-fact, many Lupus patients have different needs.

For me, finding out I have Lupus was tough. Going through the different phases of Lupus was/is challenging. Taking all the medications for Lupus seemed worse than the disease! Some say that a cure for Lupus is just around the corner. If doctors can treat it and put it back into remission, then the cure for it must be close behind? If you want to go somewhere fast, go alone. If you want to go somewhere far take others. Please join my voice and let's rise up against this disease and remember the shoes you put on today may not be the shoes you will be wearing tomorrow.

If this book has helped just one person become more aware, at ease, or has helped with their diagnosis of Lupus, then all my hard work has paid off. Please feel free to contact me with any questions. You can reach me via e-mail at amendrin@yahoo.com

Thank you,

Allen Mendrin

ACKNOWLEDGEMENTS

I would like to thank the following people who have helped, encouraged, inspired and loved me through this process: My beautiful wife Nicole and our precious dog Lola, my mother Carolyn, sister Stephanie and her husband Jeff (and the kids Jillian, and Kayden,) my sister Susan, my brother Michael, my father-in-law Jeff and awesome mother-in-law Lisa, Jordan, my grandmother Verna and grandfather George, Nicole's grandparents Jeanie and Marvin, the many doctors and the many others who have prayed, supported and helped guide me through this process.

Thank you, I love you all!

www.ingramcontent.com/pod-product-compliance
Lightning Source LLC
Chambersburg PA
CBHW050808290526
45792CB00001B/36